Assertive outreach
in mental health

....

Peter Ryan

DPSW, MPhil

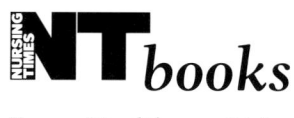 *books*

Emap Healthcare Ltd
Greater London House
Hampstead Road
London NW1 7EJ

Nursing Times Clinical Monographs are authoritative, concise, single subject publications designed to provide a critical review of material that will be of value to practising nurses, midwives and health visitors. Their authors, all experts in their field, are asked to be challenging and thought-provoking and to stimulate reflection on current practice. *Nursing Times* Clinical Monographs do not seek to be exhaustive reviews but up-to-date overviews; their critical and evaluative nature is designed to promote best practice through consideration of current evidence.

Topics for publication are decided by the editorial advisory board, with input from practitioners. Monographs are then commissioned as near as possible to the publication date to ensure that the information they contain is the latest available. All manuscripts are reviewed by a board member and a clinician working in the field covered.

At regular intervals, 12–15 new monographs will be published. They will cover subjects suggested by practitioners (see below) and any major new developments in the field of nursing care. Each publication will be on sale for a limited time, after which it will be withdrawn and, if necessary, replaced with an updated version.

Note: For referencing purposes NT Clinical Monographs should be treated as books

Suggestions for future titles are welcome and should be sent to Simon Seljeflot at NT Books, Emap Healthcare, Greater London House, London NW1 7EJ

Study Hours
All NT Clinical Monographs have been given a Study Hours rating. This is an approximate guide to the amount of time it might take a nurse, midwife or health visitor with no specialist education on the subject to read and reflect on the article and consider the suggested key reading list. By doing this you can accrue Study Hours to help towards your PREP study acitivities. Make a note of any related study you undertake and keep a record in your personal professional profile. For your free Study Hours pack, call 01483 455040.

The Study Hours logo is a registered trade mark of Emap Healthcare Ltd.

Assertive outreach in mental health

Peter Ryan, DPSW, MPhil

The government has decided to make assertive outreach a central feature of its new mental health policy. Mental health service users fear that it may affect their civil liberties, but mental health service providers are under pressure to implement it. There is, however, considerable ambiguity around the term itself, about which model is most effective, and what skills and resources are required to implement it. This monograph seeks to provide a brief overview of assertive outreach and covers definitions and models of assertive outreach, policy context, the target group for assertive outreach, the ACT model of assertive outreach, research evidence for the efficacy of the ACT model and implications for practice

Definitions and models of assertive outreach

One of the difficulties is that there is enormous variation in how the term is defined. In the UK, the Labour government has used the term 'assertive outreach' in its white paper *Modernising Mental Health Services: Safe, Sound and Supportive* (Department of Health, 1998).

The new National Service Framework also uses the term assertive outreach. However, in mental health policy and research literature a number of terms are used almost interchangeably. These include assertive community treatment, clinical case management and intensive case management. For the purposes of this monograph, these terms are regarded as equivalent to the term assertive outreach.

However, a number of different models or approaches of assertive outreach have evolved and developed, particularly in the USA. These include the strengths model (Rapp, 1992, 1998), the rehabilitation-oriented model (Anthony et al, 1993), clinical case management (Roach, 1993) and

assertive community treatment (ACT) (Stein and Test, 1980). However, it is important to note that the ACT model has been evaluated far more extensively than any of the others and for this reason has gathered a greater degree of empirical validity. The model that will be focused on in this monograph will be ACT.

In a useful overview, Onyett (1992) defined assertive outreach as 'a way of tailoring help to meet individual need through placing the responsibility for assessment and service coordination with one individual worker or team'.

This emphasises the fact that a central feature of assertive outreach is that it both coordinates and individualises care. The care needed by individual clients is carefully and comprehensively assessed, leading to a tailored and unique package of care for each. This can be done either through one individual being specifically responsible for delivery of the care package or for a team as a whole to share responsibility for the effective coordination of care.

One of the central defining aspects of assertive outreach is the context in which it occurs, and the kind of client to whom it is offered. These important aspects of assertive outreach are highlighted in the government's own definition (Department of Health, 1998) as follows: 'Assertive outreach is an active approach to treatment and care for those who are at risk of being readmitted to psychiatric hospital. Such people are typically hard to engage because of their negative experiences of statutory services. Assertive outreach . . . ensures that treatment is delivered early enough to prevent the patient's condition from worsening.'

This definition highlights the proactive nature of assertive outreach and the fact that it is designed to operate on the client's own territory in the community; it is not an office-based service. It reaches out to the client rather than expecting the client to reach out to it.

Assertive outreach, therefore, can be very effective in engaging high-risk clients with complex needs who otherwise might have fallen out of contact with services. Equally, assertive outreach is designed to avoid unnecessary hospital admissions and therefore it assists clients to stay in the in the community, which is where the great majority of them wish to stay.

However, the government's definition leaves out a number of essential features. For example , it talks of 'preventing the patient's condition from deteriorating'. This is very much a minimalist definition of the rehabilitation potential of assertive outreach. It misses out a central feature: its function of enhancing the psychosocial functioning of clients, optimising their quality of life and assisting them in recovery.

Through the delivery of high-quality psychosocial interventions to clients their capacity can be restored to an optimal level. This integration of engagement, care coordination and psychosocial rehabilitation is the distinctive feature of the ACT model of assertive outreach.

In summary, assertive outreach is an approach to care that :
● Engages high-risk severely mentally ill clients with complex needs who are resistant to contacting services;
● Proactively reaches out to clients in their own territory in the community;
● Assesses need comprehensively, develops individually tailored care packages and effectively coordinates care across agencies;
● Optimises the rehabilitative potential of clients by delivering clinical interventions that enhance client functioning.

Policy context

The Conservative government's reforms 1990–1997

The mental health field has seen more policy change and development in the 1990s than during any comparable 10-year period. Both the Conservative government and the Labour administration saw mental health as a field requiring major policy reform. Because of this, mental health services have been in a constant state of upheaval and restructuring from 1990 onwards.

In 1991, the Conservative government restructured the way in which mental health services were organised by introducing the care programme approach (Department of Health, 1990). This was designed to ensure that the care in the community of all clients leaving a mental hospital would be effectively coordinated by ensuring multidisciplinary discharge planning and by appointing a nominated key-worker to coordinate each client's care package.

In 1993 social services were restructured to ensure that they targeted care at the most vulnerable and severely disabled clients, assessed need on an individually tailored basis and monitored the delivery of an appropriate care package on a costed basis. Both these reforms were undertaken with a view to enhance the coordination and efficiency of care in the community. Importantly, both health and social services were given a fixed annual budget within which to operate. There was to be no 'bailing out' by central government if this budget was overspent.

The requirement of efficiency, bringing with it the pressure to control and reduce costs, had somehow to be reconciled with other policy requirements. At the same time, the Conservative government was introducing reforms such as the purchaser/provider split, the individualising of care delivery through needs-led assessment and the involvement of users and carers in the planning and management of services.

The 1990s also saw the closure of mental hospitals at an unprecedented pace, leading to the rapid reduction of hospital beds. Inevitably, demand for this decreased number of beds has been rising, and the number of admissions consequently has risen steeply, from 200,000 in 1983 to 270,100 in 1994–95 (Sainsbury Centre, 1998a). This meant that the newly implemented administrative systems of the care programme approach and care management were under pressure to coordinate care of an increasing number of patients who were being discharged into the community with increasing frequency.

Around the mid-1990s public concern over the safety of care in the community rapidly escalated as a result of a number of tragic incidents in which members of the public or of the caring professions were killed by patients with severe mental illness 'at large' in the community. The incident that received most press coverage was the murder of Jonathan Zito by Christopher Clunis in 1992 (Ritchie, 1994).

This led to the establishment of a supervision register under the care programme approach in order to monitor the behaviour of high-risk clients more closely. In addition, new legislation was enacted in order to the make the supervised discharge order available to mental health services. Essentially, supervised discharge made it possible for mental health services to call a review under the care programme approach for clients who caused major concern and to make their return to hospital more readily and speedily available.

Under the Conservative government the overall balance of community care policy tipped much more explicitly towards the close monitoring and control of high-risk clients, particularly those likely to be violent.

New Labour's approach: the 'failure of community care'

This concern with the public safety aspects of care in the community has gathered pace under the direction of the Labour government. On July 29, 1998, health secretary Frank Dobson drew a line under community care for people with a mental illness, saying that a 'third way' had to found. The new policy initiative had to reconcile supporting people in the community with enabling them to be recalled to safer, more restrictive environments when there was evidence that there was a threat either to their own safety or to the community at large.

The white paper: Modernising Mental Health Services (1998)

This has set out the Labour government's vision of how it wishes mental health services to develop over the next 10 years. A package of new measures has been announced which is designed to balance extra support with greater security for the public. It includes the following:

● Assertive outreach teams to engage with and monitor at-risk mental health services users;
● Secure units in each region for the most seriously disturbed clients;
● A 24-hour help-line and crisis intervention teams to respond to emergency needs;
● Extra acute in-patient care beds, hostels and supported accommodation;
● Clear guidance on the most effective drugs and therapies to be provided by the National Institute for Clinical Excellence;
● The establishment of home treatment teams;
● A national service framework for standards of care.

The new mental health policy is summarised as follows (Department of Health, 1998): 'People with mental health problems often have complex needs that cross traditional organisational boundaries. A modern mental health service will provide care that is integrated and focused on the individual, recognising that different people have different needs and preferences. It will be evidence-based and outcome-driven. Services will be there for people when they need them and where they need them. Services must be safe, sound and supportive. Partnerships will be crucial.'

The title 'safe, sound and supportive' is worth closer scrutiny. It encapsulates the essence of Labour's 'third way' approach. It strikes a new balance between public safety on the one hand and the right of service users to receive 'sound, supportive' services on the other.

Underlying the concept of 'safe' services appears to be a high level of confusion and ambiguity. The initial statement refers to a duty of mental health services as a matter of first priority to 'protect the public'. Subsequent statements refer initially to the safety of 'patients, service users, carers, the staff and the public'. So whose safety actually comes first? Where are services to place priorities?

Consequences for assertive outreach
It seems clear from the white paper (Department of Health, 1998) that the primary task and role of mental health services will be that of protecting the public. In many ways, this seems more radical than anything undertaken by the Conservative government. These pressures towards an increased emphasis on prioritising public safety must give some cause for concern to mental health service providers. The government clearly sees assertive outreach as a means of establishing service contact with and tracking and monitoring high-risk and potentially violent clients.

This control aspect of assertive outreach is of particular concern to service users. There is a risk that user perceptions of services, and of assertive outreach in particular, may change. Users could be forgiven for becoming more cautious and more reluctant to engage with services that might be required, at a crisis, to prioritise public safety above user concerns. Thus, paradoxically, the increased emphasis on public safety may have a negative effect on another aspect of policy outlined in the white paper: making services more accessible to users and increasing engagement.

The target group for assertive outreach

Who are the most appropriate clients for assertive outreach? In terms of service costs, this group can be characterised as 'high cost/low volume'. It has been estimated that this relatively circumscribed group of people in need of intensive support accounts for 80% of the direct costs of mental hospital treatment and care for people with schizophrenia. A recent report (Sainsbury Centre, 1998b) concluded that assertive outreach was the treatment of choice for the most problematic of the severe long-term client group.

In overall terms, the prevalence of this group is likely to vary considerably from as high as 200 per 100,000 in an inner city to as low as 14 per 100,000 in rural areas. The report estimates an average prevalence of 45 per 100,000 or a maximum of 15,000 nationally.

Some of this group may be causing anxiety or concern in their local communities through their history of violence against others; many more will be at risk of suicide or severe self-neglect. To put this in perspective, about 50 homicides and 1,000 suicides per year are likely to involve people with long-term severe mental illness (Appleby, 1997).

Many clients in this group will have experienced frequent readmissions to inpatient care or extended periods of time of a year or more as inpatients. Some may be caught up in the judicial system as minor offenders, while others might be homeless or frequently change address. Many others may be experiencing problems with drugs or alcohol as well as long-term mental illness.

A recent study (Ryan, 1999) found that more than 80% of clients on the caseloads of the assertive outreach teams had at least one of the following criteria: history of self-harm, history of

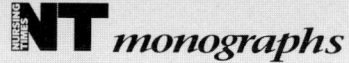

violence, non-compliance with medication, non-cooperation with mental health services or at least one admission in the past two years.

The clinical process: the ACT model of assertive outreach

Historical context

In 1970, Leonard Stein took up the post of director of education and training at Mendota State Hospital in Madison, Wisconsin, USA. Working together with his long-term colleague Mary Ann Test, Dr Stein began to develop what in the early 1970s was a radical departure in the kind and quality of care in the community for clients with long-term mental illness. He wrote: 'We decided to change the focus of our efforts from activities in an inpatient setting designed to prepare the patients to live in the community to activities in an outpatient setting designed to help patients make a sustained adjustment to community life' (Stein and Test, 1992).

They developed an intensive community support programme for psychiatric inpatients who had proved difficult to discharge and called it total in-community treatment. They had concluded that these patients had several features in common which were independent of diagnosis: a limited range of instrumental and problem-solving skills, strong dependency needs and heightened vulnerability to stress.

Stein and Test (1992) hypothesised that the community would be a better location than the hospital for treatment of these problems, because it was more likely to require and reinforce appropriate behaviour and to present good role models of individuals coping adequately with living in the community. It would also provide a precise focus for skill training in the particular locations where adaptive behaviour was required.

After much negotiation Stein and Test managed to secure the agreement of hospital administrators to redeploy hospital ward staff in the community. Instead of being based on an inpatient ward, staff were located in an old house in Madison. Staff coverage was available 24 hours a day, seven days a week.

An individually tailored treatment programme was devised for every patient, based on an assessment of their deficits in the coping skills necessary for independent living in the community. In essence, staff would do whatever necessary in order to keep the patient out of hospital.

Most treatment took place *in vivo*, in patients' homes, neighbourhoods and places of work. The focus was on training patients in the specific skills necessary in their particular living situation to survive adequately in the community. This meant that patients were assisted to use the particular gas cooker, or washing machine, or bus route they needed to manage in order to adjust to their particular niche in the community. In addition, patients were given sustained and intensive assistance in finding a job or sheltered workshop placement.

Staff would remain in contact afterwards, in order to help resolve any problems that might emerge once a job had been started. Patients were also assisted in exploring their use of leisure time and in the development of effective social skills.

Stein and Test (1992) tried to build on the strengths and competencies of clients. They worked with the patient's family; where the ties with the family were pathological, they would encourage 'constructive separation'. They would work with friends and neighbours who might be providing additional support. They engaged in assertive outreach in the sense that, if a patient initially refused to see the case manager, they would persist in their attempts at engagement. They would assess the patient's need for medication and ensure that medication compliance was adhered to. Hospital inpatient facilities were used very much as a last resort.

National and international expansion of the ACT model

The bold innovations in treatment developed in the ACT model have led

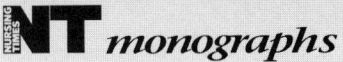

Notes

to enormous interest, both in the USA and internationally. The positive results obtained through rigorously conducted research evaluations enhanced the burgeoning reputation of the approach. Programmes borrowing heavily from the ACT model are now found throughout the USA (Bond, 1995).

The ACT model has received considerable attention overseas. Hoult and his colleagues set up and evaluated an ACT programme in Australia (Hoult et al, 1984). In the late 1980s, a team based at the Maudsley Hospital, London, developed and evaluated the daily living programme, which again was largely based on the ACT model (Muijen et al, 1992).

Aims of ACT
Allness and Knoedler (1998), in a comprehensive overview of the ACT model, defined its aims as follows:
● To lessen or eliminate the debilitating symptoms of mental illness each individual client experiences and to minimise or prevent recurrent acute episodes of the illness;
● To meet basic needs and enhance quality of life;
● To improve functioning in adult social and employment roles and activities;
● To increase community tenure;
● To lessen the family's burden of providing care

Selection criteria
Allness and Knoedler (1998) summarised selection criteria for ACT as follows:
● Clients with severe and persistent mental illness, with priority given to people with schizophrenia, other psychotic disorders (for instance, schizoaffective disorder) or bipolar disorder;
● Clients with significant functional impairments with respect to at least one of the following: difficulties in daily living skills; finance management; repeated evictions or loss of housing; difficulties in sustaining daytime occupation;
● Clients at high risk of self-neglect or harm to self or others;
● Clients with coexisting substance

misuse of significant duration (for instance, more than six months);
● Clients with high use of acute psychiatric inpatient care (for instance, two or more per year) or of psychiatric emergency services.

How, operationally, might an assertive outreach team recognise such clients? Witheridge (1991) and Stein and Diamond (1985) developed the following typology of needs:

● **Unwillingness or inability to attend or keep appointments for services**
Many patients with severe and persistent mental illness are unwilling to seek treatment. Some simply do not wish to attend appointments under any circumstances, while others attend infrequently and often miss appointments. Such clients have traditionally been labelled 'unmotivated' and therefore not fit for treatment. Stein and Test (1980) took the bold and imaginative step of developing the strategy of assertive outreach, whereby the programme would go to the client, rather than the client to the programme.

● **Need for direct assistance in coping with daily living**
Clients requiring ACT are likely to need help with the most basic details of everyday life — cooking and cleaning, negotiating for and cashing their welfare benefits cheque, shopping for food, getting around on public transport, and so on. Budgeting and managing their money may be another area where they might need assistance.

● **Need for medication**
Stein and Diamond (1985) stated their position quite clearly: 'Patients who are not willing to take their medications on a regular basis require a treatment approach that can monitor them very carefully and use a wide variety of incentives to ensure that they take needed medication.'

● **Assistance with housing**
Clients are likely to need help in acquiring and maintaining decent, affordable accommodation, whether that is in the private rented sector,

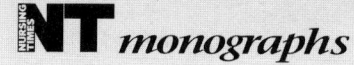

local authority housing or specialist housing support.

● **Need for structured daily activity**
Some patients are likely to need help in finding meaningful, productive day-time activities. For some this may mean actively seeking work, for others developing a pattern to their day-time activity so that their time is occupied in a way that is meaningful and satisfying.

● **Ability to self-monitor symptoms**
Patients vary considerably in their ability to recognise an increase in their own symptomatology. Where patients are aware of this they are likely to appreciate the need for professional assistance in order to avoid relapse and readmission. More intensive follow-up is required where patients are unaware of an increase in symptomatology or resist professional assistance.

Staffing and organisation
The ACT model adheres to the following staffing and organisational patterns (Allness and Knoedler, 1998):
● Small caseload (client/team member ratio of 10–15:1);
● Regular review of care plan for each client;
● Team leader is a practitioner with a caseload;
● Continuity of staffing;
● Psychiatrist on staff (client/psychiatrist ratio of 100:1);
● Multidisciplinary staff mix, with a core of nursing, social work and occupational therapy staff, with sessional input from clinical psychology;
● Skill mix includes capability for behavioural/family intervention, early-signs monitoring and medication adherence;
● Substance abuse specialist on staff (50:1 ratio);
● Employment rehabilitation specialist on staff (100:1 ratio);
● Community support workers on staff;
● Team consists of at least 10 full-time members.

Organisational boundaries
● Explicit admission criteria;

● Intake rate of six clients per month or fewer;
● Full responsibility for treatment services;
● Responsibility for hospital admission;
● Responsibility for crisis services/24-hour cover;
● Responsibility for hospital discharge planning;
● Service not limited to specific time periods.

Working hours of most assertive outreach services are flexible and include seven-days-a-week, 24-hour availability. The model requires a multidisciplinary team approach, including the sessional input of psychiatrists and clinical psychologists and the full-time input of community psychiatric nurses, social workers, occupational therapists and community support workers. As indicated above, caseload size needs to be low, no more than 1:10–15.

Service values and principles
The principles of ACT can be summarised as follows:

● **An assertive approach**
Lack of motivation and social withdrawal are frequently observed aspects of the secondary ongoing effects of schizophrenia. This creates a dilemma for office-based community services, since clients with long-term mental health problems are often not very good at turning up at the office and keeping appointments. For this reason, traditional community services often have trouble keeping in touch with long-term clients.

Stein and Test (1980) were among the first to emphasise the critical importance of assertive outreach. They pointed out that, although there was a fine line between assertive outreach and infringing on the civil liberties of clients, it was perfectly possible to respect the client's rights while still doing far more than traditional approaches in reaching out to the client.

They wrote: 'When we find the client we don't hit him over the head, shanghai him and haul him back to

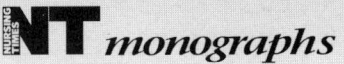

Notes

the programme; but we do stop him, talk to him and try to convince him that we would really like to get re-involved with him. The patient may say no the first few times we try, but in our experience he will eventually come back into the programme. This approach has markedly reduced drop-outs from our programme.'

● *In vivo* **services**
The rationale for delivering *in vivo* services is well summarised by Stein and Test (1985): 'To begin with, skills learnt in a natural setting can be used later with little or no additional require-ment to generalise. Thus, unlike skills learnt in institutional settings, such as hospitals or day centres, skills learnt *in vivo* can immediately begin to make a difference in the actual living environ-ment of the client.'

Skill development is carried out in the environment where the client is actually encountering problems in adaptation. Hence he or she can be encouraged to develop coping skills in the precise location where they are likely to be of most benefit.

● **Retaining responsibility for patient care**
Coordination of the many services required for people with a long-term mental illness is an essential require-ment. Traditionally, this had been done through good will and good co-operation. Stein and Test (1980) com-mented: 'Although referral and interagency communication are neces-sary, they are not sufficient; the key-stone to coordinated services is a fixed point of responsibility so that, even though there are many agencies pro-viding services, one remains responsi-ble to see that all those services are delivered. Assertive outreach was developed to do that job.'

● **Provision of material resources**
Stein and Test (1980) recognised that an effective programme of community support had to start with ensuring that the client had access to the basic mate-rial resources required to survive in the community — food, shelter, clothing, and so on. The secret was to ensure that each individual client acquired the particular set of resources he or she needed. In addition, these had to be delivered to clients in a way appropri-ate to their particular setting in the community.

● **Development of coping skills to meet the demands of community life**
A whole variety of skills are required to adapt and live in the community, such as self-care, cooking, budgeting money, using public transport and so on. Traditionally, these skills had been taught in hospital rehabilitation pro-grammes, only for both staff and patients to discover that they did not translate effectively to the settings in the community where they had to be exercised. It was far better, therefore, to develop these skills *in vivo*, where they had to be put into practice.

● **Motivation to persevere and remain involved in life**
Stein and Test (1980) found, as had many others, that patients were highly sensitive to the stresses of everyday life in the community. They would often react by rapidly losing their capacity to cope effectively, their motivation to survive in the community apparently much reduced.

Unlike many others at the time, they did not blame the patient for being poorly motivated. Rather, they developed a system of care, ACT, which would provide 'a readily avail-able system of support to encourage the client, to help him solve real prob-lems and to help him feel that he is not alone and that others are concerned about his welfare'.

● **Optimising the home environ-ment**
Stein and Test (1980) defined a difficult home environment as 'one which inhibits personal growth, reinforces maladaptive behaviour and generates feelings of panic in its members when its loss is threatened'. They recognised that such relationships could occur both in hospital and in the commu-nity. This might imply working with families to optimise family communi-

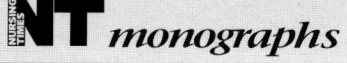

cation and support or, where this is not possible, to assist the client in finding an alternative living environment.

● **Titrated support**

This principle recognised that patients need ongoing support in the community but that the amount of support required may vary considerably. The task of a treatment programme was to be sufficiently responsive and flexible to deliver to the patient the appropriate level of support: neither too much nor too little.

● **Relating to patients as responsible citizens**

Stein and Test (1980) commented that '[relating to patients as responsible citizens] is extremely important for staff in order to work effectively with patients as well as with the community. Staff must believe that the people they are working with are citizens of the community, that they are living in the community because they have a right to, and not because the community, through its good graces and kindness, is allowing them to be there; that they are indeed free agents able to make decisions and be responsible for their actions.'

● **Crisis intervention available 24 hours a day, seven days a week**

One of the important innovations engineered by Stein and Test (1980) was to extend the concept of 'normal working hours. They stated: 'These patients don't limit their crises from nine to five, and hospital admissions generally are over-represented after five at night, at weekends and on holidays — periods of time when the normal support system is unavailable. Twenty-four-hour-per day availability of a crisis response ensures that a support system is always available to the patient.'

● **A team approach**

An important feature in the ACT model is a team approach. Its advantages are as follows: first, a team approach maximises the likelihood of continuity in the delivery of services,

in that if one worker is on leave, or sick, another can take over. Secondly, a team approach can increase the creativity available to develop care plans. Thirdly, it can maximise the chances to avoid burn-out as well as encouraging the development of staff morale.

Witheridge (1991) put this point well: 'The burdens of the work become ours, not just mine, and the accomplishments — including those that might seem inconsequential to outsiders — likewise belong to everyone.'

As far as the UK is concerned, there has been much emphasis on individual responsibility and accountability. Through the key-worker role in the care programme approach, it is necessary to mitigate the total team approach as practised in some ACT services in the USA.

Allocation of individual key-worker responsibility is necessary under the care plan approach. This ensures a specific allocation of responsibility, while enabling the team to deploy a variety of team members to deliver aspects of the care package to the individual client, including specific psychosocial interventions.

Skills and functions of ACT: the integration of 'core skills' with psychosocial rehabilitation

The model emphasises the assertive outreach team as a primary provider of many of the services required by the client. This involves the combination of core skills and functions in an integrated holistic manner with key rehabilitation functions. This is outlined in Table 1 overleaf.

Its approach is comprehensive, covering not only mental health and rehabilitation needs but also basic material survival needs, such as housing, food and health care. Its direct service provision includes medication, long-term one-to-one therapeutic clinical relationships, 24-hour crisis availability, family support and intervention, early intervention to prevent hospitalisation, orientation towards daytime

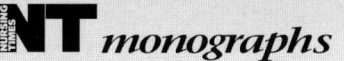

Table 1. The integration of core skills and psychosocial rehabilitation in ACT

Core skills
Engagement
Non-office based community outreach
Comprehensive, needs-led assessment
Care planning
Linkage with community resources (housing, social security)
Maintenance and expansion of social networks
Collaboration with in-patient services and prevention of hospitalisation
Advocacy
Monitoring and review

Psychosocial rehabilitation skills
Early intervention and symptom management
Behavioural family intervention
Cognitive behavioural intervention
Assistance with daily living and occupational skills

---

occupation, services and assistance with housing and daily living skills.

Core skills and functions of ACT

Perhaps the central feature of the core functions of an assertive outreach team is that it has to be prepared to work on the clients' own territory and to be persistent in trying to contact them in responsive, practical, client-centred ways.

In this model, comprehensive need assessment is crucial (Allness and Knoedler, 1998). This involves the following:
● Client strengths, aspirations and resources, including an account of vocational, educational and social interests;
● Psychiatric history, status and diagnosis, including assessment of presenting symptomatology, perhaps through systematic assessments, such as the Brief Psychiatric Rating Scale (Overall and Goreham, 1962);
● Housing and living situation;
● Self-care abilities;
● Family and social relationships, including assessment of social functioning, perhaps through systematic scales. such as the Life Skills Profile (Rosen et al, 1989);

● Family education and support needs;
● Physical health;
● Alcohol and drug misuse;
● An understanding of the gender, ethnic and racial aspects of need assessment.

Clinical interventions with respect to these core functions include the following:

Direct assistance with meeting basic needs
Staff from the team help clients meet basic needs for adequate shelter, food and health care in ways that maximise community integration and enhance patient satisfaction. Whenever possible, accommodation is in 'normal' housing rather than in specialist mental health housing facilities. Staff visit frequently to assist clients *in vivo* to develop the appropriate coping skills.

Assistance with a supportive social environment
Staff also focus on assisting patients to develop their own network of family and friends, as well as providing, through their own relationship, a secure source of support. They also run discussion groups and psychoeducational programmes.

Notes

Psychosocial rehabilitation skills and functions

A comprehensive series of supporting psychosocial rehabilitation services are offered to the client through the same team.

Early intervention and symptom management

Minimising psychotic symptomatology and the prevention of relapse is given high priority. Specific interventions include identification of early warning signs and relapse signatures (Birchwood et al, 1998), continuous monitoring of appropriate levels of medication, 24-hour crisis availability and occasional brief hospitalisation.

Behavioural family intervention

The team often provides ongoing education to both clients and their families into the nature and management of long-term mental illness. Behavioural family interventions (Fadden, 1998) are used in order to optimise communication and support in the family. Essentially it is a form of individually tailored psychoeducational programme which seeks to preserve the family as an asset and resource to the patient. The programme attempts to facilitate supportive but not over-involved or destructive relationships with the patient and the family.

Assistance with daily living and occupational skills

Rather than allocating the client to homogenous sheltered workshops, the team places great emphasis on developing an individualised occupational plan for each patient. Often this involves part-time work or encouraging a leisure activity.

Clients are taught the appropriate occupational skills for the appropriate setting and are also supported through any difficulties they might encounter in the work setting. Employers are helped to understand the difficulties the client may be encountering, are themselves supported through any anxieties or concerns they may be experiencing and are also encouraged to structure the work environment to make it more responsive to and accommodating of the client.

The research evidence

The ACT model of assertive outreach has received extensive evaluation. What follows is a brief overview.

The classic early Madison study (Stein and Test, 1980)

This was not only one of the earliest attempts to evaluate the efficacy of assertive outreach, but arguably one of the most successful. The study was carried out in two major stages.

During the first stage, which lasted 14 months, patients were randomly allocated either to ACT community treatment or to a control programme consisting of standard hospital and community care.

In the second stage, the ACT intervention was stopped and the effects of reintegrating the ACT patients into standard community care evaluated. All patients were aged between 18 and 62 and had any diagnosis other than primary alcoholism or severe organic brain syndrome.

Over the first stage of 14 months, when the experimental group was receiving ACT, only 18% were hospitalised for a mean of 11 days. The re-admission rate was under 10%.

The results for the control group were strikingly different. Here, 88% were hospitalised, with a readmission rate of 60%. Also, inpatient length of stay was much longer, at an average of 36 days. There were also significant differences in favour of the experimental group in terms of reduction in symptomatology, higher levels of employment, a greater number of social relationships and higher patient satisfaction with quality of life.

Striking as these results are, Olfson (1990) advised interpreting them with caution, since a lower proportion of the experimental group were diagnosed with schizophrenia (50% compared to 79%), and rather more had an acute illness, thus giving greater potentiality for improvement.

In the second 14-month period, when the experimental group was

Notes

reintegrated into standard community care, all the gains made began to deteriorate. There was a gradual increase in hospital use, social relationships declined in quality, symptomatology increased, time spent in sheltered employment declined and overall satisfaction with quality of life decreased.

Concerning the deterioration in evidence during this second period, Stein (1992) commented: 'What this experiment made clear is that we need to move from a time-limited model to a model that provides services indefinitely. In retrospect it seems obvious that when we deal with an illness that we do not know how to prevent or cure, and that is thus chronic in nature, the intervention must likewise be long term in nature.'

International replication of the ACT findings

The first major international replication of the ACT model came from Hoult and his colleagues, who set up an ACT service in North Shore, Sydney, Australia (Hoult et al, 1984). Their target group were mixed-diagnosis, difficult-to-treat patients who were assigned at inpatient admission either to the experimental programme or to standard inpatient care. They were comparable to the patient group treated by Stein and Test (1980).

Results at the end of the first year indicated much reduced hospital inpatient care (a mean of 8.4 days compared to 53.5 days for the control group). Programme costs were also significantly less.

On one outcome measure, the experimental group was less symptomatic than the controls, although on others there were no differences; they were also more satisfied with their care and had higher psychosocial performance. There were no differences in occupational outcome, although it should be noted that this was the area which was least comparable to the ACT model.

Somewhat disturbingly, 10% of patients in the experimental programme made attempts at suicide, compared to none in the controls.

An overview of recent research on assertive outreach

Both the original research carried out by Stein and Test (1980) and the international replication carried out by Hoult et al (1984) produced a comprehensive array of positive results. The length of stay in hospital and the number of hospitalisations were reduced; community tenure was increased and clients stayed for longer periods of time in their accommodation in the community; symptoms were reduced and overall level of psycho-social functioning increased; clients perceived their quality of life as having improved and much preferred assertive outreach to standard services.

Since the early 1980s, when these studies were carried out, numerous evaluations on assertive outreach have been undertaken. What follows is an overview of some of these more recent studies.

Engagement

Two UK studies found very high levels of engagement. Ford et al (1995) found that 95% of clients receiving assertive outreach were still in contact with services over an 18-month period, while Thornicroft (1998) found that no clients at all who were receiving assertive outreach were lost to care during the 18 months of his study.

Reported engagement levels in the USA, while still high, have been somewhat lower than these. Bond et al (1995), in a meta-analysis, found average engagement levels of 75%. On the other hand, a recent UK study found that more clients lost contact with their worker in low caseload services compared to high caseload services. (Burns et al, 1999).

Hospitalisation

In the USA, Bond et al (1995) found average reductions of 50%. Also in the USA, Mueser et al (1998) found that, of 23 studies that examined hospital bed use, 14 reported significant reductions in length of stay.

Two UK studies have produced interesting results. The Daily Living Programme (Muijen et al, 1992; Marks et al, 1994) used a prospective clinical

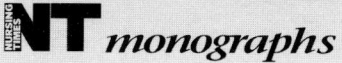

Notes

trial design. Patients with severe long-term mental illness were randomly allocated either to standard inpatient care, or to the Daily Living Programme (DLP), which was closely based on the ACT model. Prevention of hospitalisation was a key treatment aim and was dependent on the DLP team retaining the authority to admit and discharge.

Reporting on the first six months follow-up, Muijen et al (1992) found that the DLP reduced hospital stay by 80% (median stay six days compared to 53 days in the control group). This shorter length of stay did not lead to large numbers of readmissions. Hospitalisation was prevented altogether for 23% of DLP patients.

The North Birmingham Psychiatric Emergency Team operated a 24-hour, seven-day-a-week service, offering home-based assessment and treatment for people at risk of acute hospitalisation and was able to achieve reductions in bed use of 50% (Sainsbury Centre, 1998b).

Three other UK studies found no significant reductions in hospitalisation (Ford et al, 1997; Thornicroft, 1998; Burns et al, 1999).

Housing stability
Mueser et al (1998) found that assertive outreach significantly increased housing stability in nine out of 12 studies where this outcome was measured.

Jails and arrests
The findings here are not impressive. Mueser et al (1998) reported that in 12 studies that measured the impact of assertive outreach on involvement with the criminal justice system, only two found reductions in time spent in jail.

Symptoms
The evidence here is mixed. Mueser et al (1998) found that among the 16 controlled studies which evaluated symptomatology, eight reported significant reductions in symptomatology.

As far as UK studies are concerned, Burns et al (1993) studied home-based multidisciplinary assessment and found no differences in effectiveness compared to control services, but lower costs. Similarly, Muijen et al (1994) and McCrone et al (1994) found no differences between a team of CPNs employing case management methods with low caseloads, assertive outreach and a standard team of CPNs. Neither Burns (1999), Ford and Ryan (1997) or Thornicroft (1998) found significant improvements in symptomatology.

Social adjustment
Results in this area again are mixed. Mueser et al (1998) found only three out of 14 studies that measured social performance as an outcome reported positive results. A recent British study (Thornicroft, 1998) reports improvements in social networks for intensively casemanaged clients.

Medication compliance
Somewhat surprisingly, relatively few studies of assertive outreach have explicitly attempted to measure medication adherence. Mueser et al (1998) could find only four studies that addressed this issue, of which two reported positive outcomes. One UK study (Ryan et al, 1999) also reported positive results, finding that levels of compliance increased on average by 16% over an 18-month period.

Quality of life
Mueser et al (1998) were able to find only a moderate affect of assertive outreach in terms of improving quality of life. Six out of 12 studies that evaluated quality of life found positive outcomes. They concluded that improvements in this area may be related to linked positive changes in hospitalisation and housing stability. All of these studies also were able to achieve improvements in hospital stay, symptom reduction and more stable housing.

Client satisfaction
Mueser et al (1998) found that six out of seven studies that evaluated this factor were able to report significantly higher levels of client satisfaction with assertive outreach services compared to standard service provision.

One UK study (Ryan et al, 1999) carried out an independent user-led evaluation. The interview schedules were designed, carried out and analysed by the users themselves. The central message of this user-controlled research, was that 'in summary, the interviews and discussions elicited an overwhelmingly positive response . . . it was seen as qualitatively different from other services and as a vast improvement. The central relationship between the service user and the assertive outreach worker, as the means of negotiating a better life in the community, was understood and appreciated. It did not always work perfectly, and could not compensate for service gaps and failures, but it was better than what went before, and its loss was feared' (Beeforth et al, 1994).

It is worth noting that both the recent white papers (Department of Health 1998a; b) emphasised the importance of user consultation in the planning and delivery of services.

Conclusions

Implications for nursing and nurse education

There is little doubt that assertive outreach will be carried out in teams that will be multidisciplinary in nature, and where nurses will carry out their duties in close cooperation with social workers, occupational therapists, community support workers, clinical psychologists and psychiatrists.

The days of uniprofessional teams of CPNs, or social workers for that matter, are over. Inevitably this will lead to an increased overlap between the roles of the different professional groups working in these teams. In due course most, if not all, team members will be able to carry out comprehensive health and social care assessments, including symptom assessment, the monitoring of side-effects and so on.

Nurses involved in community care of people with mental health problems will no doubt continue to maintain their specialist role, however defined, but inevitably this will continue to narrow. It may well be that CPNs and CPN training will have a limited future.

On the other hand, skills and expertise previously possessed by other professional groups will increasingly become available to nurses. Post-registration and postgraduate courses offering these skills on a multidisciplinary basis are expanding rapidly. The opportunities for nurses to expand their role, expertise and competence are, therefore, enormous.

In due course it will be nurses who most commonly engage in early intervention, cognitive behavioural or family intervention, medication adherence or motivational interviewing. There is no doubt that nurses will continue, both numerically and in terms of expertise, to be the core professional group in terms of provision of community care for people with mental health problems. Paradoxically, they are likely to achieve this most effectively by expanding the range of their generic expertise, rather than narrowly defining themselves as professional specialists.

None of this implies the end of the various professional groups as we know them. The Sainsbury Centre's *Pulling Together* report (1997) neither recommended nor implied the merging of the professional groups into a common pool of community care workers. It does, however, imply at the post-qualifying level a pooling of skills and expertise to form the 'core competencies' recommended in the report. Nurses, more than any other professional group, have most to gain from this.

Implications for practice
Assertive outreach is not so much the treatment of choice as the only viable mechanism for ensuring that a highly vulnerable at-risk client group can be engaged in services and responded to in a needs-led manner. It prevents clients from falling through the net and ensures that they receive an appropriate, individually tailored network of services.

Assertive outreach is about far more than engagement. A 'brokerage' approach that essentially engages clients, links them to services and coordinates care may well succeed in

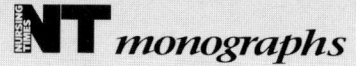

obtaining high engagement levels and some reduction in hospital admission. However, the rehabilitation potential of the client is unlikely to be realised and improvements in psychosocial adjustment or quality of life are unlikely.

Marshall et al (1997) concluded that this 'brokerage' form of assertive outreach 'does not produce clinically significant improvement in mental state, social functioning, or quality of life . . . in summary, therefore, it is an intervention of questionable value, to the extent that it is doubtful whether it should be offered by community psychiatric services.'

The ACT model of assertive outreach which integrates care coordination and psychosocial rehabilitation is more likely to optimise service gains, such as engagement and reduction in hospitalisation, with clinical gains such as reduction in symptomatology. Medication compliance can also be improved and the living situation of clients in the community can be stabilised. Under these favourable conditions, quality of life may also be enhanced. Equally importantly, clients like and value assertive outreach as a form of service delivery and usually prefer it to standard care.

The importance of effective implementation

Although all these outcomes are achievable, it has to be conceded that many of the recent UK studies have not convincingly demonstrated this. One reason might be implementing the ACT model in a systematic, thorough and comprehensive manner. It is worthwhile noting that the DLP study, which paid much attention to implementing the ACT model, also obtained, by UK standards, a relatively positive set of results (Marks et al, 1994).

In contrast, a recent study (Burns et al, 1999) focused primarily on manipulating caseload size, rather than developing the skill content of the model. The study found no differences in outcome between control and experimental conditions and concluded: 'Energy and investment should concentrate on the specific content of care (particularly that derived from evidence-based practice) rather than its form and delivery, if improvements are to be achieved.'

Assertive outreach is now a central feature of the national service framework for mental health and is in the process of being implemented on a national scale. It is crucial that the ACT model is effectively implemented.

A recent research overview of 34 ACT research studies (Latimer, 1999) found that well implemented programmes reduced hospitalisations by 58% over one year, compared to poorly implemented programmes. This suggests that it is the effectiveness with which the ACT model is implemented which determines the quality of outcomes obtained.

Methodologies are now available (Teague and Bond, 1998) to monitor the effectiveness of implementing the ACT model. We have, at last, the capability to ensure the effective implementation of this form of care.

Drawbacks to assertive outreach

It has also to be acknowledged that there are certain drawbacks and disadvantages to assertive outreach. First, it has to be remembered that assertive outreach teams are required to work with clients with complex multiple disabilities who are likely to be a high risk either to themselves or to others.

This task, while challenging and rewarding, can also be highly stressful and anxiety-provoking. Unless good systems of clinical supervision are in place, staff will themselves be at risk of burnout.

Secondly, the social control aspects of assertive outreach should not be overlooked. The government has already make it clear that protection of the public will be a high priority for assertive outreach teams.

Assertive outreach could, therefore, quite easily find itself caught in an impossible dilemma: attacked by the public and the media for not protecting the public sufficiently well, and criticised by user groups for undermining their civil liberty and cutting short their tenure in the community. **NT**

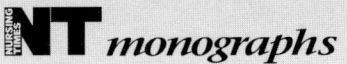

References

Allness, D.J., Knoedler, W.H. (1998) *The PACT Model of Community-based Treatment for Persons with Severe and Persistent Mental Illness: A Manual for PACT Start-Up.* Richmond, Va: NAMI.

Appleby, L. (1997) *National Confidential Enquiry into Suicide and Homicide by People with Mental Illness: Progress Report.* London: DoH.

Anthony, W.A., Forbes, R., Cohen, M.R. (1993) Rehabilitation-oriented case management. In: Harris, M., Bergman, H. (eds) *Case Management for Mentally Ill Patients.* London: Harwood.

Beeforth, M., Conlan, E., Grayley, R. (1994) *Have We Got Views for You.* London: Sainsbury Centre for Mental Health.

Birchwood, M., Todd, P., Jackson, C. (1998) Early intervention in psychosis: the critical period hypothesis. *British Journal of Psychiatry*; 172: supplement 33, 53–59.

Bond, G., McGrew, J., Fekete, D. (1995) Assertive outreach for frequent users of psychiatric hospitals: a meta-analysis. *Journal of Mental Health Administration*; 22: 4–16.

Burns, T., Creed, F., Fahy, T. et al (1999) Intensive versus standard case management for severe psychotic illness: a randomised trial. *Lancet*; 353: 2185–2189.

Burns, T., Beadsmore, A., Bhat, A. (1993) A controlled trial of home-based acute psychiatric services. *British Journal of Psychiatry;* 163: 49–54.

Department of Health (1990) *The Care Programme Approach for People with a Mental Illness Referred to the Specialist Psychiatric Services (HC (90)23/LASSL(90)11).* London: DoH.

Department of Health (1998a) *A First-Class Service: Quality in the New NHS.* London: DoH.

Department of Health (1998b) *Modernising Mental Health Services: Safe , Sound and Supportive.* London: DoH.

Fadden, G. (1998) Family intervention in psychosis. *Journal of Mental Health*; 7: 2, 115–122.

Ford, R., Beadsmore, A., Ryan, P. (1995) Providing the safety net: management for people with a serious mental illness. *Journal of Mental Health*; 1: 91–97.

Ford, R., Ryan, P. (1997) Labour-intensive: how effective is intensive community support for people with long-standing mental illness? *Health Services Journal*; January 23: 26–29.

Holloway, F. (1998) Intensive case management for the severely mentally ill: a controlled trial. *British Journal of Psychiatry*; 172: 19–22.

Hoult, J., Reynolds, I., Weekes, P. et al (1983) Hospital versus community treatment: the results of a randomised controlled trial. *Australian and New Zealand Journal of Psychiatry*; 17: 160–167.

Latimer, E. (1999) Economic aspects of assertive community treatment: a review of the literature. *Canadian Journal of Psychiatry*; 44: 443–454.

Marks, I., Connolly, J., Muijen, M. et al (1994) Home-based versus hospital-based care for people with severe mental illness. *British Journal of Psychiatry*; 165: 179–194.

Marshall, M., Gray, M., Lockwood, A. (1997) Case management for people with severe mental disorders. In: Adams, C., Anderson, J. (eds) *Schizophrenia Module of The Cochrane Database of Systematic Reviews.* Oxford: Update Software.

McCrone, P., Beecham, J., Knapp, M. (1994) Community psychiatric nurse teams: cost-effectiveness of intensive support versus generic care. *British Journal of Psychiatry*; 165: 218–221.

Mueser, K., Bond, G., Drake, R., Resnick, S. (1998) Models of community care for severe mental illness: a review of research on case management. *Schizophrenia Bulletin*; 24: 1, 37–73.

Muijen, M., Marks, I., Connolly, J., Audini, B. (1992) Home-based care and standard hospital care for patients with severe mental illness: a randomised controlled study. *British Medical Journal*; 304: 749–754.

Muijen, M., Cooney, M., Strathdee, G. (1994) Community psychiatric nurse teams: intensive support versus generic care. *British Journal of Psychiatry*; 165: 211–217.

Olfson, M. (1990) Assertive community treatment: an evaluation of the experimental evidence. *Hospital and Community Psychiatry*; 41: 634–641.

Overall, J., Gorham, D. (1962) The brief psychiatric rating scale. *Psychological Reports*; 10: 799–812.

Onyett, S. (1992) *Case Management in Mental Health.* Cheltenham: Stanley Thorne.

Rapp, C. (1992) The strengths perspective of case management with persons suffering from severe mental illness. In: Saleebey, D. (ed)*The Strengths Model in Social Work.* New York: Longman.

Rapp, C. (1998) *The Strengths Model: Case Management with People suffering from Severe and Persistent Mental Illness.* Oxford: Oxford University Press.

Ritchie, J., Dick, D., Lingham, R. (1994) *The Report of the Inquiry into the Care and Treatment of Christopher Clunis.* London: HMSO.

Roach, J. (1993) Clinical case management with severely mentally ill clients. In: Harris, M., Bergman, H. (eds) *Case Management for Mentally Ill Patients.* London: Harwood.

Rosen, A., Hadzi-Pavlovic, D., Parker, G. (1989) The life skills profile: a measure assessing function and disability in schizophrenia. *Schizophrenia Bulletin*; 15: 325–337.

Ryan, P., Ford, R., Beadsmore, A., Muijen, M. (1999) The enduring relevance of case management. *British Journal of Social Work*; 29:

Notes

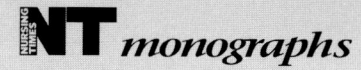

97-125.

Sainsbury Centre for Mental Health (1997) *Pulling Together: The Future Roles and Training of Mental Health Staff.* London: Sainsbury Centre for Mental Health.

Sainsbury Centre for Mental Health (1998a) *Acute Problems: A Survey of the Quality of Care in Acute Psychiatric Wards.* London: Sainsbury Centre for Mental Health.

Sainsbury Centre for Mental Health (1998b) *Keys to Engagement: A Review of Care for People with Severe Mental Illness Who are Hard to Engage With Services.* London: Sainsbury Centre for Mental Health.

Stein, L., Test, M. (1980) Alternatives to mental hospital treatment: conceptual model, treatment program and clinical evaluation. Archives of General Psychiatry; 37: 392–397.

Stein, L., Test M. (1982) Community treatment of the young adult male patient. *New Directions for Mental Health Services*; 14: 57–67.

Stein, L., Diamond, R. (1985) A programme for difficult-to-treat patients. In: Stein, L., Test, M. (eds) *The Training in Community Model: A Decade of Experience.* San Francisco, Ca: Jossey Bass.

Stein, L. (1992) Innovating against the current. *New Directions in Mental Health*; 56, 5–40.

Teague, G., Bond, G. (1998) Program fidelity in assertive outreach: development and use of a measure. *American Journal of Orthopsychiatry*; 68: 2, 216–232.

Thornicroft, G. (1998) The PRISM psychosis study articles 1–10. *British Journal of Psychiatry*; 173: 363–431.

Witheridge, T. (1991) *The Active Ingredients of Assertive Outreach: New Directions for Mental Health Services.* San Francisco, Ca: Jossey-Bass.

Recommended reading

Allness, D.J., Knoedler, W.H. (1998) *The PACT Model of Community-based Treatment for Persons with Severe and Persistent Mental Illness: A Manual for PACT Start-Up.* Virginia: NAMI.

Birchwood, M., Todd, P., Jackson, C. (1998) Early intervention in psychosis: the critical period hypothesis. *British Journal of Psychiatry*; 172: supplement 33, 53–59.

Department of Health (1998) *Modernising Mental Health Services: Safe, Sound and Supportive.* London: DoH.

Mueser, K.T., Bond, G.R., Drake, R.E., Resnick, S.G. (1998) Models of community care for severe mental illness: a review of research on case management. *Schizophrenia Bulletin*; 24: 1, 37–73.

Sainsbury Centre for Mental Health (1998) *Keys to Engagement: A Review of Care for People with Severe Mental Illness Who are Hard to Engage With Services.* London: Sainsbury Centre for Mental Health.

Notes

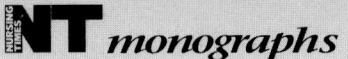

Notes

Notes